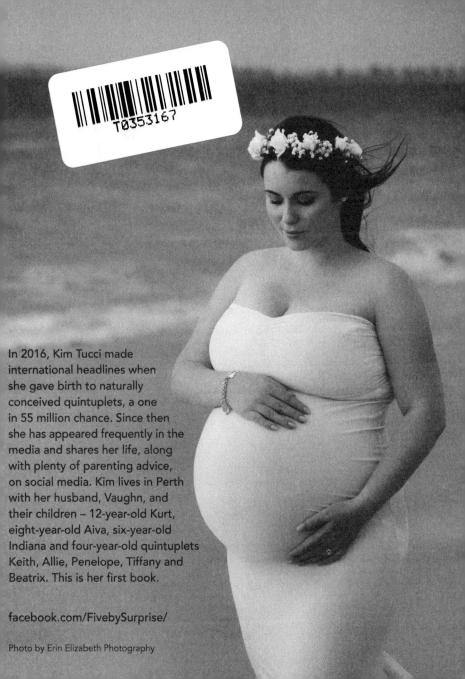

In 2016, Kim Tucci made international headlines when she gave birth to naturally conceived quintuplets, a one in 55 million chance. Since then she has appeared frequently in the media and shares her life, along with plenty of parenting advice, on social media. Kim lives in Perth with her husband, Vaughn, and their children – 12-year-old Kurt, eight-year-old Aiva, six-year-old Indiana and four-year-old quintuplets Keith, Allie, Penelope, Tiffany and Beatrix. This is her first book.

facebook.com/FivebySurprise/

Photo by Erin Elizabeth Photography

I've had 8 babies, and if there's one thing I've learned ...

150+ tips for all new parents to save sanity, time and money

Kim Tucci

Australia's Quintuplet Mum

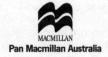

MACMILLAN

Pan Macmillan Australia

For Michael White, who believed in me when I didn't believe in myself.

You are always missed.

Contents

Introduction

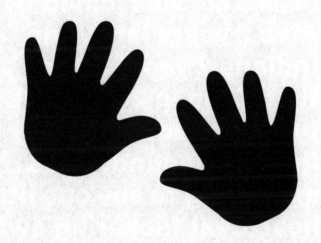

I became a mum to Kurt at 17; I was a kid having a kid. At 19 I met my husband Vaughn, and little Kurt was joined by Aiva 2 years later, and Indiana 2 years after that. Then in 2015, I fell pregnant again. At the first ultrasound, I was expecting to see one little heartbeat flickering away. When I saw five strong heartbeats, I couldn't even begin to imagine what my life would look like in the future.

Preparing to welcome five babies into our family home was not an easy task. Emotionally, I had to do some serious soul-searching to find the courage and strength required to manage a high-risk pregnancy. And on a practical level, it seemed almost impossible. For a start, we needed five times the amount of everything – nappies, clothing, bottles, bassinets, bedding, car seats – just for the first weeks alone!

Nothing could have prepared us for becoming a family of ten. To be honest, before Keith, Allie, Penelope, Tiffany and Beatrix arrived, I had been pretty much making up parenting as I went along. I certainly didn't appreciate the importance of establishing good sleeping habits until I had five babies sleeping at different times of the day and night. With the quintuplets' arrival, I needed to find a better way not just to survive, but to thrive. Because, yes, I am a mother – but first and foremost I am Kim, and I want to be able to enjoy each day with my beautiful children without waiting for bedtime from the moment I wake up!

So, this book contains some of the practical tips and tricks I have learned along the way to make life easier for myself and my family, covering everything from meal times with babies and toddlers, encouraging good sleep habits, tear-free bathing and stress-free toileting; to creative ideas for rainy-day play, having the best fun on a budget and how to clothe your kids without breaking the bank – all while making time for some much-needed self-care, too.

I hope this book helps to make your parenting life a little simpler, a little cheaper and a lot more fun.

Kim

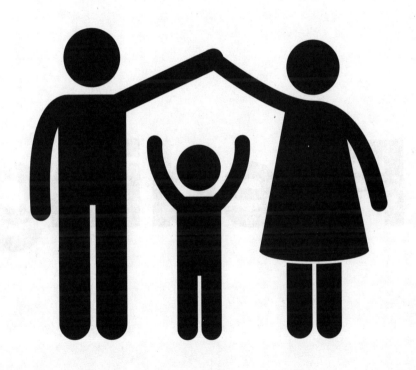

Feeding

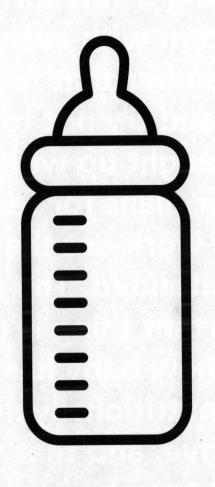

Feeding a newborn is different with each baby. Remember that fed is best and try not to get too caught up with worry if your plans for feeding don't work out the way you intended. The most important thing is that your new baby has what they nutritionally need to thrive, and that you aren't too stressed out in the process!

Don't be afraid to ask your midwife for help before you are discharged from the hospital. Midwives have a wealth of knowledge and can offer excellent advice – mine gave me formula and bottle recommendations for the quintuplets. Many midwives have undergone training as lactation consultants or can organise for a specialist to visit you before you are even discharged from hospital.

Try breastfeeding your baby in the bath. The skin-to-skin contact helps release oxytocin to help you and your baby relax and to promote let-down.

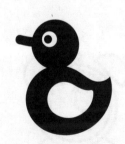

Newborns will need to feed every 2–4 hours, but the time is actually measured from the beginning of one feed to the start of the next. This means that if it takes 30 minutes to feed your baby, they might be ready for another one 90 minutes later. (Maternal and child health nurses will generally encourage you to try to space feeds to 3–4 hours so that your baby is hungry enough to drain both breasts properly and get both the sugary foremilk and the creamier hindmilk.)

Set up a breastfeeding station. There is nothing worse than waking up in the night to feed your newborn, only to find you need something that is out of arm's reach. Here's what I had in my breastfeeding station:

- A warm blanket in winter or a fan for hot sticky nights

- The TV remote or book/magazine

- A pillow to support my arm when feeding

- Extra bibs or cloths

- Nipple cream

- A bottle of water.

Invest in a comfortable maternity bra and some stretchy tees. You don't need to buy lots of expensive nursing tops. A few key pieces of maternity wear will see you through. Washable cotton breast pads will save on extra costs, and they're absorbent and gentle on the skin.

Lactation cookies are a delicious way to boost your milk supply. They are packed with nutritious ingredients, such as brewers' yeast, wheat germ, flaxseed and whole oats. Lactation cookies can be bought online – or you may be lucky enough to have a friend who loves baking and is keen to make a batch for you! The herbs milk thistle and fenugreek have also traditionally been used to promote milk supply. You can buy them as capsules or in drink form from health-food stores.

To soothe grazed, sore or cracked nipples, squeeze some breast milk out after feeding and gently rub it over the nipple – the antibodies and vitamins in the milk will help repair the skin. You can cool the inflammation with a frozen kitchen sponge placed in a zip-lock bag, or freeze some breast pads dampened with cold water and use those (also in a zip-lock so you don't 'burn' your skin).

Put refrigerated cabbage leaves in your nursing bra – as strange as this sounds the leaves have an anti-inflammatory effect and help soothe sore breasts. I have tried this, and it works a treat!

Breast milk will keep up to 6 months in the freezer, so don't be afraid to freeze it. Some extra-clever trays are designed to freeze the milk in long blocks, which you can then transfer to a bottle to thaw. I asked my midwives for some milk-storage containers to take home that were compatible with my breast pump. There are also disposable milk bags available in most chemists that are a good solution for freezing batches of milk.

If you're struggling with your supply, consider donated breast milk. If, like me, you give birth to more than one baby, or you're experiencing difficulties with your supply, this is definitely something to consider. Milk banks are heavily monitored and there are strict screening protocols to check for infectious diseases, alcohol, smoking and medication use. (Donors have blood tests every 90 days to check for these.)

When introducing breast milk in a bottle, try and do it when you're not in the room. Chances are if you are around the first time, bub will fuss for the comfort of the breast. Be patient and gentle; don't worry if this process takes a while – it's a new learning curve for your little one too, and every baby is different. Be consistent, and eventually the bottle will be taken.

Set up a designated bottle station. It makes life so much easier. It's a good idea to keep your bottles all the same brand and type because, before you know it, you can forget what part goes with what bottle! Set aside a clean area in your kitchen and assemble everything you need for the station. Here's what my feeding station had:

- Formula

- Clean bottles (start with two bottles and see how you go)

- A 2-litre jug with a lid, filled with boiled water cooled to a warm temperature

- A clean container with dummies ready to go if required after a feed

- A bottle-drying rack. Make sure you buy one that's easy to clean as they can attract mould if not washed and dried often enough.

Sometimes it can take a bit of trial and error to find a bottle teat that your baby likes. You may need to try a few different brands until you find the right one.

For bottle-feeding when you're out and about, take a bottle filled with cooled water from the kettle. You can buy a container for the formula, or a small zip-lock bag is much cheaper and just as convenient. Don't forget to pack a spare formula scoop from one of your finished tins.

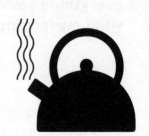

A bottle holder can make life much easier. Sometimes you might need a little extra help if you have older children running around when you're trying to feed your bub. I had an amazing little pillow that looked like a bib with a bottle holder stitched into it. It was my little lifesaver at feeding time!

At night, a bottle warmer can come in handy if you aren't keen on microwaving or waiting for a bottle to warm up in a sink of hot water. I used a formula-making machine for the quintuplets. It made a nice warm bottle, and all I had to do was press a button and give the bottle a good shake!

Dream feeding – feeding your baby while they are asleep – is possible whether your baby is breastfed or formula-fed. This saves you from having to go through the process of nappy-changing and resettling. Gently pick your baby up and bring them to the breast or bottle – they will instinctively attach even though they are sleeping. Ideally, you will feed your baby just before you go to bed to ensure that you're getting a long stretch of sleep throughout the night before the next scheduled feeding. Use a night light or other very dim light so you don't mess with your bubba's body clock (or your own).

Don't feel bad when someone tells you their newborn is 'sleeping through the night' when you and your baby are up at all hours. All it means is that their baby is able to sleep from around midnight (or the time of the last feed) to about 5 am – which I'm told is not all that common, especially for breastfed babies. (Breast milk is generally easier for babies to digest, so their tiny tummies are likely to need a refill sooner than formula-fed infants.)

To avoid falling asleep with the baby in your arms, set your phone alarm to vibrate after 5–10 minutes. That way you can wind your baby and then gently pop them back in the bassinet or cot.

Let your partner share the night feeds. If you're someone who does not do well without sleep, put some plans in place so you don't end up a complete wreck. This might mean, for example, expressing and letting your partner or other caregiver do one of the night feeds.

FED IS BEST

When it comes to feeding babies, I've pretty much experienced it all. My first child, Kurt, was born 6 weeks premature. I would express beside his humidicrib in the hospital so I could smell him and hear his cry, as this always helped with let-down. My second baby, Aiva, took to the breast and it all came very naturally. I fell pregnant with Indiana when Aiva was 13 months old and I was still breastfeeding her. I slowly weaned her throughout the pregnancy. I had every intention of breastfeeding Indi for as long as I fed Aiva, and had no reason to expect that I couldn't, but my body had other ideas. I tried pumping every few hours with an electric breast pump as well as latching Indi onto the breast, but I wasn't producing more than 30 ml from both breasts at a time. I felt like an absolute failure, and Indi went onto formula by the time she was a week old. I was so worried this meant I wouldn't bond well with her or that she might be missing out on important nutrients. I look back at that time and realise how hard I was on myself. Indi not only survived but thrived! She was happy, healthy and robust. At the end of the day filling that tiny belly with nourishment is all that matters. Yep. Fed is best.

When your baby is ready, you can introduce solids – usually at 6 months, and not before 4 months. Keep it simple – there's plenty of time in the future to try exciting new foods and recipes.

Introduce one food type at a time to detect any intolerances or allergies. I would always start with simple foods, such as mashed potato, and only introduce one new food every few days.

Try pureeing single vegetables first, such as potato, carrot, pumpkin or broccoli. Store them in an ice-cube tray and pop out the portions as you need them. This will prevent any food spoilage, and save time and money. Making your own baby food means you know exactly what's in it, plus it's cheaper and avoids heaps of jars and plastic ending up in landfill.

Reusable squeeze pouches are both eco-friendly and cost-effective. They are easy to wash, dry and refill, plus you can keep them in the freezer.

Mesh feeders can be filled up with fresh fruits and given to a teething baby who has sore gums. A friend brought around five mesh feeders, and they were a godsend! Not only were the symptoms of teething relieved, but I had five quiet babies who were happy to munch away on delicious fruit juices, and I didn't have to worry about choking because the fruit was contained inside the mesh pouches.

After trying individual veggies, start to mix them or add little portions of each to meal time. If all is going well with feeding and you haven't experienced any issues or reactions, try adding some small pieces of meat, such as cooked mince.

USE SILICONE BIBS.

I had a massive pile of cloth bibs in the early days. They would quickly get smelly from milk and food stains required soaking after meal times. Before I knew it, we were washing 20-plus bibs a day! I was gifted five silicone bibs when the quintuplets were around 6 months old; I still have the same bibs, free from stains and in good knick after 3 years of use!

Start to offer finger foods when your baby is between 7 and 10 months. Go for soft or well-cooked foods in small pieces to avoid a choking hazard. Here's a list of first foods you can try:

toast fingers

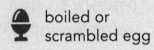 boiled or scrambled egg

grated cheese

sliced banana

sliced avocado

pasta shapes

diced watermelon

sliced ripe pear and stone fruit

cooked corn kernels

steamed broccoli and cauliflower florets

sliced cooked pumpkin, potato and sweet potato

diced cucumber

At 12 months, your baby can enjoy the same foods as the rest of the family. Try offering bite-sized portions of whatever you are eating (within reason) so that your little one can experiment with lots of different tastes and textures.

··

For safety reasons, always stay with your baby when they are eating. Make sure grapes and cherry tomatoes are cut into tiny pieces, and avoid hard or undercooked vegetables and meat that might present a choking hazard.

Try letting your toddler serve their own food with tongs. This supports independence and can help with fine motor skills. It will also prevent the plate from being overfilled with food that won't be eaten.

DON'T WORRY IF THEY DON'T EAT

I have eight children, and if there is one thing I have learned at meal times, it's that sometimes children don't want to eat and other times they don't stop eating. Don't be worried if your child stops eating; I can assure you a hungry toddler or child will eat if they are hungry. If you are concerned, keep track of your child's growth to make sure they are putting on enough weight. Most maternal child health nurses will tell you that it is completely normal for toddlers to have wildly fluctuating appetites and food preferences. Rather than worrying about what they have eaten over a 24-hour period, we should look at what they have eaten over 3 days. I remember how stressed I felt on the rare occasions that Kurt wouldn't eat his dinner when he was 2 years old. I sincerely believed that if I wasn't able to get something into his stomach it was a form of child abuse. Honestly, what was I thinking? If you have served a few different foods on the plate and they reject it all, don't resort to making a different meal to please your toddler. If a child is hungry they will eat what's in front of them, it's as simple as that.

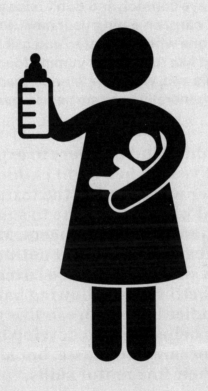

Try to remain calm if your child throws food on the floor or refuses to eat. Don't get mad, laugh or even make a big spectacle about the situation; just take the food away for the moment and take a nice deep breath. Don't make any eye contact, and don't raise your voice, just carry on eating your meal. Praise your little one when they stop and ask if they would like to eat their yummy food now. Stick to this and, with persistence, meal times will generally become hassle-free.

Allow babies and toddlers to explore food. I've watched eight children discover what food is, the texture of it and what it feels like to squish it through their little fingers. Meal times can be messy, but nothing beats a smiling baby face covered in spaghetti sauce! Allowing babies and toddlers to explore in this way not only helps them to develop their sense of smell and taste, but also their fine motor skills.

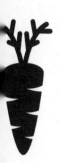

Consider a veggie boost. I use a powdered vitamin supplement in my children's meals to boost their veggie intake when I am worried they aren't taking in enough healthy food. I also use supplements in winter to help boost little immune systems.

Introduce new foods with familiar ones. Include a small portion of the new food along with a larger portion of something tried and loved. That way if the new food is refused, your toddler is still getting a decent meal. Also, don't give up. Research has shown that a food may need to be offered 12–15 times before a toddler likes and accepts it. Be patient and keep offering healthy food choices.

Eat as a family. It can be tempting to put a toddler in front of the TV with a plate of finger food, especially when you're feeling stressed about how little they seem to be eating (and you want 5 minutes to yourself). Don't do it. Even if it's just you and your little one, try to sit down to eat together. Families who eat together are happier and healthier (there's heaps of research on this). Also, eating in front of the TV means they are not only shovelling in food without noticing its flavour and texture, but also not paying attention to whether they are feeling full – behaviours that may contribute to weight issues in later life.

Don't overload the plate. When you all sit down to a meal together, give your toddler a small portion of whatever is being served. If too much is given at once, they are more likely to play with the food or start throwing it around. You can always keep the rest in a bowl with some tongs and top up your toddler's plate as they eat.

Children under the age of 5 only need water and milk to drink. There are so many baby juice products sitting on the supermarket shelves it's not funny. The added sugar in processed juice, cordial and soft drinks is not only unhealthy for a maturing gut and the first sets of teeth but they also have no dietary purpose for an adult, let alone a child.

Place a cloth or old sheet under the high chair. In the early days, I was so sick of having to clean up the mess and spills that would accumulate under the high chairs that I started putting down an old bed sheet to catch any of the mess that would fall during meal times. (Of course, if you have a pet dog, you can always call them in to clean up! Our labrador, Jemmy, loves to 'vacuum' up anything that finds its way onto the floor.)

It's not the end of the world if your children occasionally have a bowl of cereal for dinner! We can't always control what happens in our lives, but we *can* be kind enough to give ourselves a break when it's due. One night every now and then won't snowball into an apocalypse. Put your feet up and for the love of all things holy look after you and your needs for a night.

TIME OUT FOR THE COOK

As a mum of eight, I have many days where everything that can go wrong does go wrong, and the last thing I want to do is cook dinner and clean a mountain of dishes and a line of dirty faces. On days like this, I put an old queen-size sheet down on the floor, Vaughn gets some chips from the local fish and chip shop, and we all watch a movie. This makes life easier as we don't have loads of washing up – just a sheet we can shake outside and then pop in the wash.

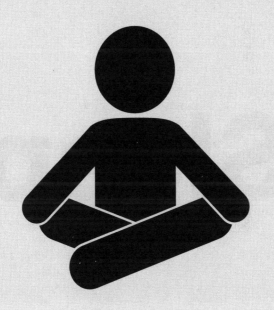

Sleep

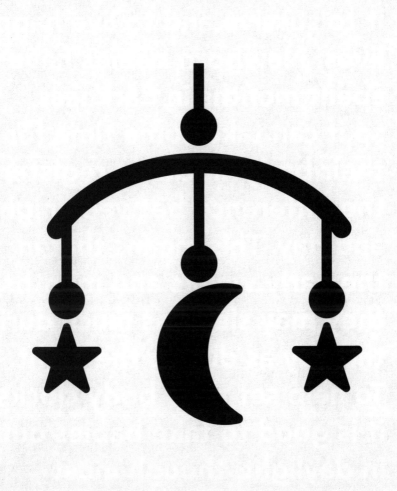

Sleep is essential – we all need it to survive and to live happy lives. Newborn babies have spent months in darkness, so it can take some time for their body clocks to register the difference between night and day. This means that in the early weeks and months, they may sleep as much during the day as during the night. To help set their body clocks, it is good to take babies out in daylight, though most newborns will be tired after

60–90 minutes of wake time. While newborns will sleep anytime, anywhere (as long as their tummies are full and they are not ill), older babies will be more sensitive to light, sound and temperature. Here are a few ways I have learned to help my babies settle at night and during their daytime naps.

Sleep when your baby sleeps, especially in the first days and weeks after your baby is born. The human body recovers while sleeping and during periods of deep sleep releases a hormone called prolactin, which assists with milk production and has an anti-inflammatory effect on the body. Think about it: your body has just gone through the astonishing task of creating and birthing a tiny human (or in my case five of them!). Be proud of what your body has achieved and allow it the rest it deserves. Sleep is also important for brain function and mood. So, sleep when you are tired and be kind to yourself, both physically and mentally.

Swaddling a baby can make them feel safe and secure. The restricted space is thought to mimic the womb, helping your baby transition to life on the outside! Try a thin muslin wrap if your baby is very unsettled – this will prevent your little one from overheating due to crying and thrashing around.

Put your baby to bed while they are tired but still awake. There will come a time when your little one will need to learn to self-settle because, let's face it, you can't be rocking your baby to sleep for the rest of their life! This doesn't mean you will need to practise controlled crying, but it is helpful if you can start to read your baby's cues and decipher if they are crying, whining or grizzling. The chances are your 3-month-old baby might be trying to self-soothe before you rush in to provide that comfort yourself. I live by the rule that if there are breaks of silence in between the grizzling, I don't enter the room. If the crying is constant, I go in to settle them, without making eye contact.

Use essential oils. Chamomile and lavender are my favourite oils for promoting sleep and relaxation in babies and children. Try them in a diffuser in the baby's bedroom or put a few drops on the edge of the 'pillow area' of the cot. Essential oils can also be used in the bath or for baby massage, although they must be diluted with baby lotion, coconut oil or olive oil.

Grab a 'helping hand'! If you're anything like me, you'll be familiar with 'dead arm' – the pain you get from resting your hand on your baby for 40 minutes while they fall asleep. Now as utterly crazy as it sounds, this trick actually does work. Place a handful of rice in a small disposable plastic glove and tie the end in a knot. Warm it in your lap for the first few minutes, then slowly replace your hand with the 'helping hand'. This keeps a comforting weight on your baby without you having to stand over the cot for hours. Stay close, though, as I wouldn't recommend leaving anything in an infant's cot unattended that might be a choking hazard. Think of this as a temporary helping hand when needed.

Keep the room cool and dark. It's always helpful to have block-out blinds to keep the room darker during daylight savings and to keep the heat at bay. I used a stick-on blind that could be attached to the window with suction cups. It was so easy to use and also portable, so if we stayed somewhere without good window coverings I knew my kids would still enjoy their afternoon nap. For a cheaper alternative, try foil: you can stick it to your window by spraying a little water on the foil first.

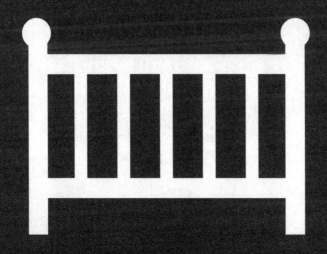

Make the bedroom a place for sleeping. Safe sleeping guidelines recommend keeping the cot free of soft toys for babies under 7 months of age. I take this a step further and keep my children's bedrooms as free from stimulation as possible. Most of their toys are in the toy room or put away in storage boxes. (Interestingly, all of the websites that provide tips for adults who have trouble sleeping suggest we keep our bedrooms free of electronic gadgets, which are our 'toys'.)

Have a sleep-time snugly toy ... and one to spare. Prepare your child for their nap or bedtime by letting them know it's just about time to go to sleep (or have 'quiet time'). Using a special cuddly toy as a signal is a nice gentle way to remind a toddler that nap time (or bedtime) will be coming up soon. It can save a lot of heartache if you invest in a backup snugly toy in case the first one gets lost. Poor Tiffany recently left her beloved rabbit at daycare and had to last all weekend without her furry friend – luckily we had a 'sister' rabbit that kept her company.

HELP WITH SLEEP

I remember visiting my GP when Indi was a few months old and tearfully asking him, 'Is it normal to be this exhausted?' He reassured me that it was all part of new motherhood and urged me to take care of myself and rest when I could. If you are struggling with sleep issues and exhaustion, there are programs that can help you cope. (Go to the Raising Children website for a list of all the public and private parenting centres in each state and territory.) There are also sleep nurses who can come to your home and support the process of transitioning from co-sleeping to independent sleeping; some even hold consultations over Skype or email. Mothers with anxiety, postnatal depression (PND) or another mental illness who are struggling to connect with their babies and/or feed and settle them can get help from a mother–baby unit (MBU) in a public or private hospital.

**Give tummies time to settle before bedtime.
A bottle of milk can be provided if under
2 years of age. Make sure food is given
45 minutes before bed to allow their stomach
to settle. This is especially important for
babies with reflux.**

••

Establish a daytime nap routine. Daytime naps are
essential for toddlers to recharge their batteries.
Research shows that they are actually tired after
2–3 hours of wake time. The key to establishing
a routine is to stick to the plan and ride out any of
the teething issues that come up in the beginning.
Now, if your toddler is unused to a daily routine,
don't worry. There will probably be tears. But
I see a big difference between a child crying
because they are starving or in pain and a child
crying because they aren't getting their own way.
The key to this is that you are making the rules,
not your children. And if having an hour or so to
yourself in the afternoons helps keep you relaxed
and happy (and makes for a more rested, happy
child!) then everyone wins.

Watch for tired signs. Tired signs can be subtle, such as rubbing eyes and yawning, or they can come in the less subtle form of tantrums – even my older children will have a meltdown if they are overly tired and don't know what they want.

I know when the quintuplets get tired they can become very clingy and want to be held, or they can become clumsy and trip over their own feet. I know my children are in need of a nap when they don't want to eat their food: it's a telltale sign in our house that it is time for bed. Get to know your own child's tired signs and it will help ensure a smoother transition to bed.

CREATING A SLEEP ROUTINE

By 9–12 months, most babies will have two daytime naps: one in the morning and one in the afternoon. And by 18 months, most will be down to just a single afternoon nap. If you keep your routine consistent, you will easily have times in the day to do what you need. For example, you might keep the morning nap time open for housework, washing or having a friend over for coffee, while you might have an afternoon nap when your little one is asleep (at least in the first couple of weeks).

Following a routine isn't for everybody, but for me it has been life-changing! I am now able to take five toddlers, a 5-year-old, a 7-year-old and an 11-year-old out of the house without being snowed under by stress and anxiety.

Here are the steps we go through for daytime naps and bedtime at night:

- - - - - - - - - - - - - - - - - - -

1. Prepare your child for their nap or bedtime by letting them know it's just about time to go to sleep (or have 'quiet time').

2. Tuck your child into bed with a cuddly toy or other comfort item (if older than 7 months) and make sure the room is cool and dark.

3. Tell your child you love them and that you will see them after their nap or in the morning.

4. Until you feel completely confident that your child is used to the routine, do not make eye contact with them. They're adept at reading your emotions, especially if you are feeling nervous about putting them down for a sleep. Those starry eyes will sense your agitation and abort the sleep mission.

5. Close the door, take a deep breath and walk away.

If one of my little ones calls out from their room, I will go in to resettle them and tuck them back into bed again. I will tell them that it is time to go back to sleep and provide reassurance if they are afraid. I always try to be firm but fair at bedtime so I know I won't be in and out of the room for hours on end. Mums and dads need a break in the evening too, so don't be afraid to be consistent with your bedtime rules.

- - - - - - - - - - - - - - - - - - -

Allow normal household noises at nap times. Whatever you do, don't creep around the house while your baby sleeps because you're afraid to wake them. Every little creak, whisper and door knock will wake a baby that has only learned to fall asleep when there is total silence. Make normal household noise at nap times and do it from the moment you bring bub home. It will help them become accustomed to the level of noise that will continue for several hours after they have been put to bed.

....

Keep pillows in place ... When the quins started using pillows at 18 months, every morning I would go into their rooms to find they had thrown all their pillows on the floor. I quickly got fed up with picking up five pillows after every sleep, so I decided to put the pillows under the sheet; this way they would stay in one spot and couldn't be moved or thrown out of the cot.

... and sleeping bags zipped up! If you are putting your child into a sleeping bag only to find it has been taken off at some point during the night (an exciting trick that can lead to extended wakefulness and other mischief), try putting the sleeping bag on backwards! That way, they can't reach the zipper (and don't worry, this is still comfortable for them).

Buy second-hand mattress protectors. The first few months after bringing a baby home is mostly filled with vomit, poo and huge piles of washing. With my first two pregnancies, I wanted the best linen, blankets and everything else a one-stop baby shop could throw at me. But when I was 27 weeks pregnant with the quins, a mum of triplets generously donated three big bags of mattress protectors. At the time I wondered if I should have bought new ones, but those protectors have been a godsend. We have five cot mattresses that are still in perfect condition after 2 years of use. No projectile vomit or poonami has ever leaked through my second-hand mattress protectors. Why buy something new if you don't have to? I have so many other things I would rather spend my money on!

Tips for quick sheet changes: I don't think any parent can be prepared for their first night-time chunder or poo explosion! One way to save yourself some time is to fold an old baby wrap or swaddle in half and place it over the top third of the mattress (securely tucking it in). The quintuplets would lay their heads over the old swaddles, which meant I only had to change the swaddle rather than a set of sheets each time one of the babies was sick – which was regularly, seeing as four of my quintuplets had reflux! Doubling up on mattress protectors and sheets means you can quickly remove a soiled top layer without the drama of changing cot and bed sheets in the middle of the night. This is another reason to be open to using preloved sheets and mattress protectors.

If you are worried about your toddler rolling out of a single bed, position a pool noodle along the edge of the bed under the fitted sheet to create a makeshift bed rail.

Make a monster spray! As their imaginations develop, it's common for toddlers and young children to become fearful of what lurks in the dark. When we moved house, Kurt was afraid of his new room. I bought a spray bottle and popped a funky-looking homemade label on it that read 'Monster Spray'. Trust me when I say that this works! Fill the bottle up with water, add a few drops of lavender oil and spray the room just before bed; don't forget to spray under the bed and in the cupboard!

Moving to a BIG BED. Most young children need very little encouragement to move into a single bed like 'big kids', especially if you make the whole experience as appealing as possible by buying some new quilt covers. Allow your child to be part of the process of dismantling the cot and setting up the new bed. In our case, logistics meant they were mostly observing, but if you can, get your toddler to help carry pieces into another room (e.g. the cot bedding). When it comes to bedtime, follow your usual routine. We made just one change: the quins could take a book to bed to look at the pictures while they were winding down and getting ready to sleep. This acted as a buffer if they were anxious and took their minds off being in a big new bed.

USING (AND SAYING GOODBYE TO) A DUMMY.

Only you can decide if using a dummy is right for your baby. While some bubs love dummies, some just aren't fussed! It can sometimes take trying a few different brands to find one that your baby likes. I used the natural rubber soothers with the quintuplets. My rule was the dummies only came out during sleep times and were not used while they were awake.

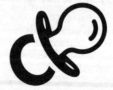

There is no easy way to say goodbye to dummies – just the thought of going through the process of getting rid of one can be daunting and guilt-inducing for any parent. Trust me I know, as I got rid of five toddlers' dummies all at once!

You may choose to tell your little one that the dummy is going to go to a new baby that needs one. You can also say that the Easter Bunny or a special fairy is going to come and take the dummy away because your child is now joining the special club for big kids. Indi never wanted to give up her bottle – I would often catch her sucking on the teat like it was a dummy. I bought her a small toy and said she could have it but she would have to throw her bottle in the bin first because she was a big girl. It worked wonders. Kurt found it really hard to break his dummy habit and it was especially tricky to wean him off it. Then one day we were at the park and he spat it out of his mouth – I just kept walking and told him it was gone now! We never looked back!

COPING WITH A CRYING BABY

1. Skin-to-skin cuddles are a great way to help calm a crying baby. Remove the clothing from the top half of your body and strip baby down to just a nappy. Find a comfortable spot and have baby lie on your chest. This has always worked a treat for my babies and dads can do this too! The sound of your heartbeat will remind baby of their time in the womb and create a soothing effect.

2. Use sheets and wraps with your scent to comfort your baby. Take some freshly washed wraps or cot sheets and sleep with them for a couple of nights. Newborns quickly learn to recognise their mother's scent, so using those sheets or wraps can have a soothing effect on your baby.

3. Try carrying your baby in a front sling (a vertical one, not one that hangs on one hip – unless you have the back muscles of an athlete!). The movement will soothe her and being close to you will help her

to feel safe and secure. If she still cries loudly, take her outside while you do some chores. The fresh air will help both of you. There are also very stylish and practical overalls called The Mumsie that are designed for baby wearing. All you need to do is pop your baby in the pouch, and off you go. I have a pair, and I absolutely adore them. I still put one of the quintuplets in at the age of 3½!

4. Know when to call time out. Persistent crying can be overwhelming, especially if you don't have anyone around to help. If you feel that you are close to breaking point, place your baby in a safe place, such as a cot, close the door and walk away for a few minutes. Babies and children pick up emotions from their caregivers, and you being frustrated and flustered makes it even harder for them to settle. Make yourself a warm drink or a snack, or call someone if you are feeling really terrible. Yes, your little one will probably continue crying, but it's important to take that break and collect yourself before you end up crying so much you need to mop the floors.

5. Don't be afraid to ask for help. Sometimes all you need is a decent sleep to give you back the energy to pick up where you left off. Call your mum, sister, aunty or a friend. And if you can't count on family or friends to step in, call your local maternal and child health nurse and they will be able to refer you to a respite program that can give you a few hours' break. YOUR welfare is just as important as your baby's.

6. Is it colic? When babies have longer crying sessions (usually an hour or more at a time) and do this more than three times a week (in the evenings), it's called colic. Now there are three important things to know about colic:

   * there's usually no identifiable medical problem that causes the crying;

   * colicky babies are perfectly healthy; and

   * the crying generally resolves by the time the baby is 3–4 months old.

7. For your own peace of mind, it's a good idea to discuss the crying with your maternal and child health nurse, or your doctor. For most colicky babies, the crying gradually builds up and peaks at about 6–8 weeks. If your baby suddenly starts crying for long periods and there has been no gradual build-up, or the crying is accompanied by other symptoms, such as a fever, consult a GP or paediatrician to rule out any other causes.

DON'T BELIEVE WHAT YOU SEE ON INSTAGRAM!

Don't compare your life with those you see on social media; I can tell you now, nothing is what it seems! Those Instagram mums who look like they always have it together generally don't – it's a charade. Try not to compare yourself to the glossy pictures of celebrity mums looking fresh-faced and ready to take on the world 5 minutes after giving birth. Those women have an army of helpers (housekeepers, nannies, personal trainers, stylists – you name it).

Nappies and Toilet Training

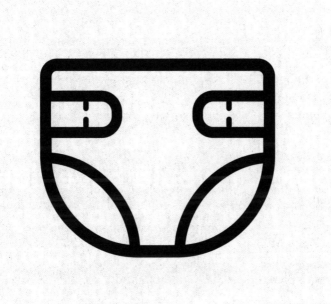

Let's talk about the nitty gritty of all things poo! Using disposable or cloth nappies comes down to personal preference. If I had been in a position to keep up with the washing and soaking of five lots of cloth nappies, I would have done it in a heartbeat: not only is it better for the environment but it saves you a fortune. If you're concerned about having to scoop the poo out of the nappy, these flushable and biodegradable.

Teaching toddlers how to use the toilet is definitely not for the faint-hearted! But we gotta do what we gotta do, right? The most important thing I've learned is that each child progresses at their own pace, and that they'll be ready when they're ready.

You can never have too many nappies. There is nothing worse than running out of nappies when you really need one. I kept a stash of nappies everywhere – in the bathroom, in my bag, in the car, even at my family's house. If you have the space, buy nappies in bulk when they are on sale and store them away until you need them.

You don't need to buy an expensive nappy bag. A backpack with a few different pockets will do the job just as well. You might want to buy a separate insulated cooler bag if you are bottle-feeding.

Consider buying preloved washable nappies. Yes, you heard that right. There is a growing market for preloved modern cloth nappies, with Facebook pages dedicated to buying and selling them. This is even better news for the environment, and a great way to make some money back on your investment.

Experiment with different nappy brands. Every baby is different in terms of shape and size, so it might take a bit of trial and error to find a brand that is the right absorbency and fit for your little one. Also, if your baby is a tummy sleeper you might find that many brands can leak overnight. If so, plastic nappy pants may help.

Don't worry too much about soaking dirty nappies. You will need a nice big bucket with an airtight lid in which to store the dirty nappies until you have enough to put through the washing machine. I don't recommend soaking the nappies in a water-filled bucket due to the drowning hazard; plus, to be honest, it gets really smelly and messy when you need to take everything out. You can sprinkle bicarbonate of soda into the pail to help with any odours – but if you are using modern cloth nappies full-time, you will need to use the washing machine every day.

**IF YOUR BABY IS SLEEPING COMFORTABLY,
YOU DON'T ALWAYS HAVE TO WAKE THEM
FOR A NAPPY CHANGE.**

**Most of the time a wet nappy can wait until
the child wakes up. Unless your little one is
prone to nappy rash or has an ulcer or some other
problem, don't stress too much about it. It's more
important that your baby is sleeping happily
(and you can also rest), rather than putting you
both through the settling process all over again.
What about poo? Most of the time it can wait,
unless it's a poo explosion, you know it will
cause upset or a rash, or it's a long time before
the next nappy change.**

Here are some simple ways to treat
nappy rash. Store-bought baby wipes
can contain irritants so it's best to use
cotton balls dipped in warm water
followed by a basic barrier cream,
such as zinc and castor oil cream.
Give baby some nappy-free time and
change nappies frequently (5–7 times
a day for babies under 12 months).

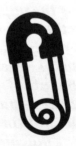

Need a secure way to prevent nappy removal? I'm no stranger to the special shock of opening a bedroom door to find a toddler has removed their nappy and there is poo everywhere. Try putting a reusable nappy cover over the nappy. If that doesn't work, the only sure-fire preventative measure (especially if it happens more than once) is to use some duct tape to secure the nappy in place. Yes, this is an extreme step but what's even more extreme is cleaning up the cot, bedding, walls and toddler who has finger-painted themselves with poo from head to toe. Yuck!

Make your own baby wipes. Have you ever looked at the ingredients on the back of your store-bought baby wipes? Some contain alcohol and a bunch of other ingredients that are too harsh for sensitive skin or nappy rash. And then there's the waste issue, since they're not biodegradable. To make your own baby wipes, all you need is an airtight container, super-soft toilet paper and water, if you want to keep it simple. You could also add coconut oil, lavender essential oil and a gentle soap such as QV to the water solution. Another option is to hem some squares of organic brushed cotton (repurposed traditional nappies are perfect) to make your own – just pop them in the container after use and put them in the wash. You can buy reusable wipe kits from online eco stores, too.

NAPPY BAG CHECKLIST

☐ five nappies (for a full-day outing)

☐ changing mat

☐ baby wipes

☐ nappy cream

☐ plastic bags for dirty nappies and wet clothes

☐ hand sanitiser

☐ two changes of baby clothes

- [ ] hat/beanie/sunscreen (depending on the weather)

- [ ] bottles, water and formula (if applicable)

- [ ] burp cloth and/or bibs (if necessary)

- [ ] breast pads (if applicable)

- [ ] a spare top for you (in case you get thrown up on after a feed, or leak through your breast pads)

- [ ] snacks and a bottle of water

If you're travelling by plane, pack one nappy for every hour. You'll likely have more than you actually need, but it's always better to prepare for the worst (a series of poo explosions/flight delays etc.) and be over- rather than under-stocked!

Use nappy-changing time to connect with your baby. As a parent, you spend A LOT of time wiping little bottoms, and these moments of one-on-one care can actually be an opportunity to connect with your child. It also helps to distract them a little if they're fidgety. Plus, talking to your little one during change time will help build language skills.

Ever wondered why there is an envelope fold on your bub's singlet or onesie? This is for when your bundle of joy has a poo blowout! You can pull the singlet down rather than up, avoiding smearing poo all over your little one's back and head. Genius, right? I only wish I knew for the first three children I had.

Watch out for the change-table wee! When Kurt was a newborn, I was changing his nappy when all of a sudden he started to wee – all over my shirt. After that experience, I always had an extra unfolded nappy on hand to block any more accidents that might come my way. I also started to watch Kurt's body language on the change table: I knew that if he had a big stretch he would be more likely to wee!

Know when your toddler is ready to use the toilet. Here are some signs that they are becoming aware of the feeling of needing to go to the toilet, or have developed enough bladder control for you both to give it a go:

- They hide in places around the house to poo or wee in their nappy.

- Their nappy is very dry, despite drinking plenty of fluids.

- They happily sit on the toilet or potty.

- They don't like the feeling of being wet or soiled.

Use books to introduce the idea in a fun way. There are some great children's books about toilet training. I found one called *Peekaboo Poo!*, which I read to the quins every night for a couple of weeks. At the end of each page I would ask, 'Where does the poo go?' And I would be met with the chorus: 'In the TOILET!' It was a fun way to get everyone used to the idea of using the toilet without it being too daunting.

Try a toddler toilet seat. I'm personally not a fan of potties. To me, it feels like double the work, as children still need to learn to use the toilet down the track anyway. Instead, I used a toddler seat that sits over the adult toilet seat, with a step and handles for safety and stability.

Clear the toilet area. It's wise to place toilet brushes, spare toilet rolls, cleaning products and anything else in a safe place out of reach of toddlers. Also, if you have a particularly inquisitive toddler (or five), have a toilet roll holder that is not easily removed (unless you don't mind fishing out a whole roll of wet paper from the toilet). If you find that your toilet starts to give off a strong odour of wee, try squirting shaving cream all over the tiled area and leave it for half an hour before wiping it up – trust me, it works!

Take toddlers to the toilet regularly. To start off, simply take your little one to the toilet about an hour after food or drink while establishing the new routine and have them climb up and give it a go. Even if your child doesn't need to go, it helps them get used to the process.

Stay calm and reassuring. Sometimes a toddler can get very upset if they want to use the toilet but are worried they can't get there in time. This learning process requires lots of praise and understanding. I know firsthand how stressful it can be when dealing with multiple toileting accidents – some days the quintuplets went through 20 pairs of undies. If you are worried about their progress, you can contact your local child health nurse for support.

Always carry a spare pair of undies, a plastic bag and wipes when you're out and about with a child who is learning to use the toilet.

A

WORD

ABOUT

REGRESSION

Sometimes, toddlers who have been successfully using the toilet for several months may start to wet their undies again. This is not uncommon, and sometimes happens when they have had a developmental spurt in another area or if they are feeling stressed. It's important not to make a big (negative) deal out of it. Instead, I bought a packet of stickers and every time the toilet was used I went out of my way to praise and give a sticker as a treat.

Bathtime and Getting Dressed

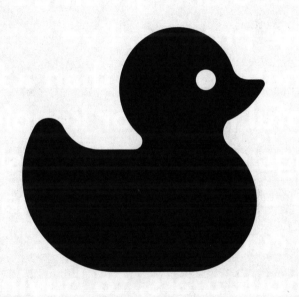

I have spent countless hours getting all eight of my children bathed, dressed and groomed. In the process, I've gathered more than a few helpful hacks for keeping things simple and hassle-free – from washing hair and cutting tiny nails without tears, to buying clothes on a budget and keeping them stain-free!

A clean laundry sink works as a bath while your baby is still small; this will save any strain on your back post-pregnancy.

Or an esky! If you are away from home and staying somewhere without a bathtub (or laundry sink), a clean esky makes a handy – and very cute – baby or toddler bath.

This is a great bathing tip I picked up from the hospital. Use a bassinet sheet over your arm to provide a better grip across your baby's back and arm when washing.

Washing toddlers' hair can be difficult. I used a bath visor hat to prevent any soap from getting into their eyes. Always make sure you have a dry washcloth nearby in case soap does find a way in.

SING SILLY SONGS AS YOU WASH. I always sing silly little songs during bathtime about each of the body parts I'm about to wash. It has turned into a family ritual now, and the kids beg me to sing the song as soon as they hear the water running in the bathroom!

Seal up bath toys to prevent mould.
If you use any plastic toys in the bath with
squeaker holes in them, seal the holes with
a hot glue gun. This will prevent any water
from getting trapped inside the toy, which
can cause mould.

Trim nails without tears! Every parent I have spoken to has a story about nipping their baby's skin when cutting their nails. I've tried everything and I swear by the Nail Snail, a 3-in-1 nail trimmer. It gives you a really firm grip and can only trim a tiny amount of the nail. I can now cut 100 nails in 5 minutes!

Add a drop of food colouring to the bath water. It creates instant fun for reluctant bathers and it won't stain the bathtub (if you don't overdo it!).

Climb in the tub with them! Your kids will love the company and it's a lovely way to bond at the end of the day.

Avoid teeth-brushing battles. Teeth brushing can be tough to start with, especially completing the recommended 2 minutes! Singing brushes and timers can help, but rather than fork out for numerous expensive electric toothbrushes, I like to sing a song about brushing teeth instead – when the song is finished they can stop brushing! I always give the toothbrushes to the quintuplets while they are in the bath or shower to help contain toothpaste mess.

Embrace preloved clothing. When friends or family offer to donate preloved clothes for your baby or toddler, accept them gratefully – anything you can't use can be passed on to charity. Better-quality items obviously last longer, especially when well cared for. Look for items such as hats, bibs, coats, shoes and dresses and pants made from hard-wearing fabric (e.g. cotton drill or denim).

Op shops are treasure troves for hand-knits. If you are a seasoned op-shopper, you'll already know that charity-run second-hand stores are full of one-of-a-kind treasures, and this is true for children's clothes, too. Keep an eye out for hand-knitted beanies, socks, jumpers and cardigans, as well as blankets for the pram or cot.

Shop at sale time. I rarely buy full-priced clothing or shoes for my kids. Instead I wait for end-of-season sales. If only larger-sized items are available, I'll put them away for next season.

·······································

Keep some clothes just for daycare. I have a box filled with dark-coloured and/or patterned shorts, pants and tops exclusively for daycare and messy play at home.

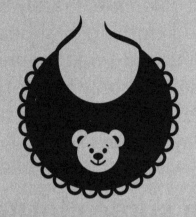

Make a bib part of your baby's outfit. There are so many cool (and comfortable) little bibs out there nowadays. Invest in a few that your baby can wear all day, not just at feeding times. Using a bib this way will keep their clothes in better shape long term, and save you a heap of washing, too.

Toddlers can be very challenging when it comes to choosing their own clothes – 'I don't want to wear THAT!' I try to set out a few weather-appropriate items of clothing the night before, and then in the morning I let them pick what they would like to wear. This usually prevents any conflict, plus setting out clothes the night before means one less thing to do during the breakfast rush. Win-win!

Help toddlers with their shoes. It can be confusing for a little one to work out what shoe belongs on what foot. I draw half a smiley face in the middle of the sole of each shoe; matching up the smile makes it so much easier to know what shoe goes on what foot.

Never lose a baby sock in the wash again! Put all your little items of clothing, such as socks and bibs, in a lingerie wash bag for safe-keeping.

Use boiling water for berry stains. If your kids are anything like mine, they absolutely love to eat berries. I always struggled to get the red and blue stains out until I found this hack. Boil the kettle, place the clothing item in the laundry sink and immediately pour the boiling water over the stain – it should lift right away!

Soak ink stains in a bowl of milk. Take the section of clothing with the ink stain, scrunch it up and place it in a bowl of milk. Rub with a dollop of dishwashing detergent and leave for 1 hour before washing. For tough stains, leave overnight.

Give rogue tissues a dose of aspirin.
If you've ever opened the door of your
washing machine to clothes speckled
with disintegrated tissues, fill a large
bucket with hot water, add four aspirin
tablets and wait for them to dissolve.
Soak the clothes in the bucket for
15 minutes and hang directly on the line.
The tissue residue will disappear in the
blink of an eye.

Keep forgotten washing smelling fresh.
Have you ever put on a load of washing
and only remembered late at night?
If it's a cool evening, put the washing
in a basket just outside the laundry.
I guarantee it won't smell at all in the
morning and it will be fresher than
keeping it in the machine all night.

First Aid and Safety

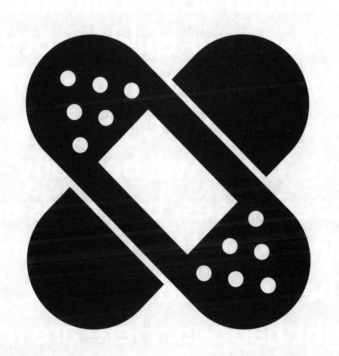

One thing I have learned as a parent is that no matter how much you would like to wrap your child in cotton wool and prevent them from ever being hurt, you just can't. There will be many grazed knees, bug bites and splinters and it's important to be prepared for what might happen. Here are my tips on surviving sick days and making your home as safe as it can be.

CREATE YOUR OWN FIRST-AID KIT

We've always made our own first-aid kits. We buy a plastic toolbox from a craft store and fill it with the following essentials:

☐ CPR guidelines for children and adults

☐ First-aid guidelines for choking

☐ Fire blanket

☐ A few clean face cloths or tea towels in a zip-lock bag

☐ Gauze in sterile packs

☐ Bandages for compression

- [ ] Fabric band-aids (Let's get real, the plastic band-aids with the cute designs always fall off as they just don't have the sticking power required for slobbery little fingers.)

- [ ] Scissors (for cutting bandages)

- [ ] Disposable gloves

- [ ] Tweezers (for splinters)

- [ ] Cold pack that activates when opened

>

- [ ] Saline (to wash out any wounds or cuts)

- [ ] Thermometer

- [ ] Rehydration sachets

- [ ] Antiseptic wipes

- [ ] Stingose

- [ ] Aloe vera gel

- [ ] Kids' paracetamol

- [ ] Kids' ibuprofen

- [ ] Sterile eye wipes and a plastic cup

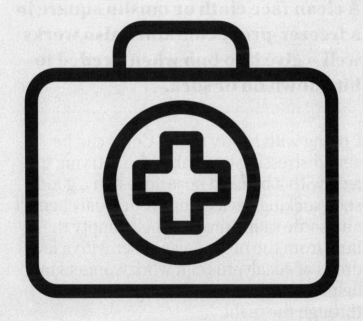

A few teething tips ... Keep teething toys in the fridge or freezer so they're cold. You can also fill a bottle teat or dummy with water and freeze them to provide relief for sore, swollen gums. A clean face cloth or muslin square in a freezer-proof container also works well – give it to bub when needed to bite down on or suck.

Coping with snotty noses. Colds can be very distressing to a baby who is trying to feed with a blocked nose. Invest in a good snot-sucking device from your local chemist and some saline drops to help empty the fluid from the nose. A vaporiser with a few drops of eucalyptus can work wonders in helping a little one with congestion sleep through the night.

When dealing with gastro, my first tip is to make sure you wear disposable gloves when cleaning up! Pop the gloves on at every nappy change and every time you clean up any vomit to prevent any germs spreading. The last thing we need as parents is to fall ill when our children are sick. It's also a good idea to have a sick bucket preprepared. You can pop in some antibacterial wipes, a face cloth and an old towel or two, so you're all ready to go when the dreaded gastro hits.

An itchy mozzie bite is surely one of the most irritating sensations, and children can't help but scratch away until their skin is red and raw. I give my children an ice pack from the freezer to help soothe the itch; this usually helps to stop their scratching. Chamomile lotion can also do the trick.

Try a bicarb paste for splinters. Make a thick paste of water and bicarbonate of soda and apply it to the area where the splinter is located. Cover with a cloth band-aid and leave it for 24 hours. After removing the band-aid, the fragment should have come out or be sticking out enough to be easily pulled out with some tweezers.

Track doses on the medicine bottle. When you've been up all night looking after your sick child, it can be hard to recall when the last dose of medicine was given, especially if you're using ibuprofen and paracetamol in tandem. Use a marker to write the time of the last dose on the medicine bottle and you (and other carers) will be able to keep track easily.

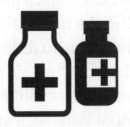

Keep little hands out of cupboards and drawers. In the absence of a child safety lock, cookie cutters and coat hangers all work, but I've found the easiest – and most discreet – solution is a simple hairband or two.

....

Attend a baby and child first-aid course. Many maternity hospitals and first-aid organisations offer hands-on courses. Before I took the quintuplets home, I went to a short first-aid session in which the midwives and doctor ran through all the basics. When Beatrix choked on a piece of meat shortly after she turned three, I knew exactly what I had to do to dislodge the food caught in her throat. A first-aid course run by qualified practitioners will teach you a range of essential skills such as this, as well as giving you more confidence as a new parent.

When your baby starts crawling, explore your house from their perspective. That's right – get down on all fours and crawl around! This is the best way to locate any potentially dangerous spots, such as power sockets, exposed wiring and any chemicals and medicines in accessible drawers and cupboards.

101 uses for pool noodles!
To prevent little fingers from being slammed or jammed in a door, cut a pool noodle in half, and then cut it open lengthways (like a hotdog roll). Enclose the vertical edge of the door in the noodle (above the handle and out of reach of little hands). This works for hinged and sliding doors. Pool noodles are also great to use for sharp corners and edges on furniture and steps.

Playtime

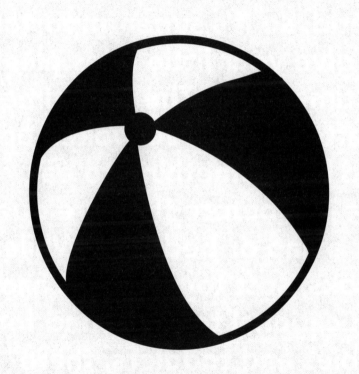

Play is how babies and toddlers learn everything about themselves and their world, so it's super important to give your little ones plenty of time for it. The best time is after they have woken up and had something to eat, not just before they are due for a nap or bedtime. While books, soft toys, blocks and educational toys abound for babies and toddlers, there are many activities you can do that don't cost a bundle, but are still loads of fun.

Play with sensory bags and bottles.
If you don't want to dabble in the messy realm of arts and crafts, then this is the activity for you. These are also really easy to make. All you need is a couple of large sealable bags or empty bottles (think large sandwich bags and disposable water bottles), then you simply squirt some different colour paints, water, rice and/or glitter into them. The bags can be laminated or sealed with clear contact paper to ensure the contents don't spill and to prevent a choking hazard. This activity can be enjoyed by all babies and children and even adults – I kid you not, it's absolutely relaxing to play with one of these as a 30-year-old woman!

Create your own road mat. Grab a large piece of cardboard and get your kids to help draw the roads, trees and buildings. You can use an old shoebox for the garage. For older children, take a large sheet of paper, some acrylic paint and a few old toy cars. Spread a thin layer of paint over the lid of an ice-cream tub or similar, roll the wheels in the paint and enjoy making tracks on the paper.

MAKE YOUR OWN PLAYDOUGH

No need for store-bought dough – it's easy to make your own. And don't worry about buying all the fancy accessories. Raid your utensil drawer and bring out your rolling pin and any plastic cookie cutters you have.
If you have any leftover cupcake liners from baking, you can use them to make dough cupcakes and cookies.
Here's a really simple recipe:

8 tablespoons plain flour

2 tablespoons table salt

3 tablespoons warm water

1 tablespoon cooking oil

a few drops of food colouring

Mix the flour and salt in one bowl, and the water, oil and food colouring in another. Pour the water and oil mixture into the flour mixture and use your hands to make a dough. Store in a zip-lock bag.

For stress-free painting, spread an old sheet or shower curtain across the floor (or deck if you're outside) and use an old shirt as a smock. Stick to one or two colours at first (avoid black). Place the paint in an old container secured to the craft table (or a board on the floor) – the last thing you want is a paint-covered missile! Supervise your toddler (unless you don't mind them doing a complete kitchen/patio makeover!).

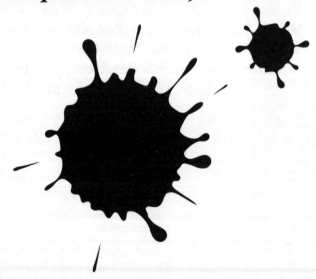

Toddlers love waterplay! Outdoors is best for this, although if you have a tiled kitchen or other waterproof area, indoors is fine, too. You just need a low table, a large plastic container and a few different-sized containers for pouring. Add a toy tea set for even more fun. Trust me, they'll do this for hours.

**Make a DIY baby pool.
Connect four pool noodles
with connectors and place over
a soft surface (grass, outdoor
playmat), preferably in the
shade. Cover the noodle circle
with a good-quality tarp. Add
water with the garden hose
(or watering can) until you
make a little 'pool' a few
centimetres deep. Get into
your bathers and splash around
together to your heart's content.
Remember: NEVER LEAVE
YOUR BABY UNATTENDED,
not even for 10 seconds.**

**GET CREATIVE IN THE KITCHEN.
Cooking together is great for
developing your toddler's fine
motor skills. Choose no-bake
recipes, such as bliss balls, that
are super easy and fun to make.
Little ones also love helping to stir
mixture, roll dough and cut out
cookies. Older kids enjoy making
pizza – encourage them to choose
and then add their own toppings.**

Make pasta necklaces.
This is a really cheap, easy
and fun activity for rainy
days – all you need is penne
pasta and some paint and
string. Kids will love painting
and then threading their own
jewellery, and it's great for
helping to develop fine
motor skills, too.

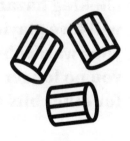

Build a cubby house. Create a secret hideout using just a sheet, a table and some cushions – and for even more fun, eat a picnic lunch in your cubby.

....

Make a dress-up box. You don't need to buy expensive superhero or princess costumes. Fill a box or basket with old clothes, hats, bags and jewellery (being careful of beads and other choking hazards) and your toddler will love playing dress-ups. Go through your wardrobe first and put in anything you no longer wear, then visit op shops for other bits and pieces.

Join the local buy, sell and trade pages on Facebook. There are so many pages devoted to baby clothing, equipment and toys where you'll find hundreds of items in great condition for a fraction of the price of new. My city also has a page for free items for those struggling financially. If you don't feel comfortable writing a post requesting help, ask one of the page admins to write an anonymous post for you. Little ones don't know the difference between new and second hand!

Rotate your toys. Fill a couple of plastic containers with toys and store them out of reach. Every few months, when the current toys are getting a little 'boring', bring out a different container. It will be like Christmas day all over again – without the price tag!

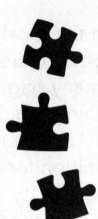

* *

Keep plastic toys clean, especially after sickness. Put them through the dishwasher every so often to keep them free from germs.

* *

Visiting a toy library is an exciting trip for a toddler that doesn't cost an arm and a leg. You can also borrow some bigger items that you may not want cluttering up the house (or at least try them out before you buy them). Many libraries will hire out stuff for parties, too! It is a great foundation for learning to respect other people's belongings. All you need to pay is a small annual membership fee and you are set to borrow away.

Make packing up toys a game. After the quins have finished playing with their toys, they all need to pack away before they take out something for their next activity. For example, they need to pack away all their books before I bring out the colouring pencils and paper to draw on. We make it a game to see who can clean up the fastest, offering lots of praise in the process. Setting a kitchen timer is also a great way to do it!

Outings
and
Occasions

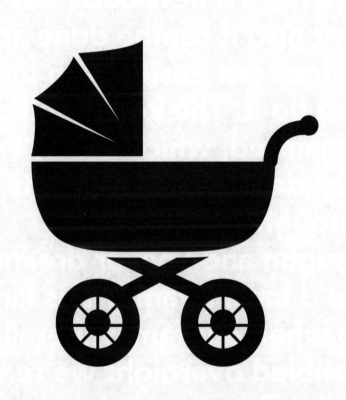

Getting out and about can be a daunting task when you have a new baby but fear not, it can be done and it does get easier each time you do it. The key is being organised, which is why I've included lots of checklists throughout this book. Vaughn and I never dreamed we'd have a family this large, so when our family literally doubled overnight we really had to learn to make our money go further. I get so many questions about how budget and still take the kids on regular outings and celebrate special occasions. Let's just say I have done my research! There are times when I don't need to live on such a tight budget, but I prefer to because I can spend any excess money on something else for the family ... or even a day out for myself!

DRIVING
WITH KIDS

Some kids love the car, and others hate it! Indi suffered from reflux as a newborn, and I was always worried she would vomit while I was driving and I wouldn't know. I bought a kids' car mirror so I could see her. If you have an unsettled baby in the car, try talking and singing to them – it sounds too simple to be true, but it does work. Sometimes when a parent is out of sight, it's reassuring for a child to be able to hear their voice. When Indi was 6 months old, I would put a slightly warmed wheat bag on her lap for extra-long car trips. The weight and the warmth of the bag provide comfort and you can add a couple of drops of lavender oil for good measure. Music works, too – there are tons of kids' playlists out there, as well as audiobooks for older children. And if your little one uses a dummy, keep a spare in a container in the car, just in case it happens to roll under the seat and out of reach.

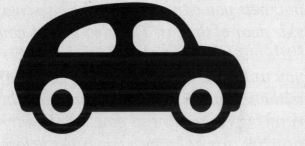

Pack the pyjamas and a fresh nappy! If you have a long drive home, put your little one in their PJs before you jump in the car to enable a smooth transition into bed.

....

For carpark safety, make a family rule that everyone who gets out of the car must hold hands. There are also handprint stickers and magnets you can attach to the passenger-side door of the car. The idea is that your little one/s keep one hand on the sticker while you unbuckle another child or get organised without having to stress about your child running rings around you. (Make sure you practise this at home a few times before going out, as it might take a few goes for them to master the art of standing still!)

How to stay sane while grocery shopping? ALWAYS have a list – the longer you take, wandering around trying to remember what you need, the more likely your little ones will become bored. Make sure they have a full tummy before you go to the supermarket, and bring some treats to give them as a reward for good behaviour when you're loading your items on the conveyer belt to pay.

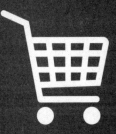

THE BOOT BAG

You never know when a vomit might surprise you or when your baby's dummy or bottle might be sneakily thrown out of the pram without your knowing. So, I always carry:

☐ a spare feeding bottle

☐ a spare dummy

☐ an old towel

☐ a few spare nappies and some travel-sized wipes (or spare undies if you have a toddler)

- [ ] a couple of books and toys

- [ ] a picnic blanket for impromptu park trips

- [ ] sunblock

- [ ] a power bank for your phone so you don't miss out on any photo moments

TAKE YOUR TIME

Sometimes it can take a while to feel comfortable going out with your new baby, especially if you have little support from immediate family, had complications with the birth, or have a premature or sick baby. When Kurt was released from the hospital (he was 6 weeks premature) I was so worried about him falling sick due to his impaired immune system that it was hard for me to leave home. I was also very young, so most of my friends were not at the point of wanting to have a family yet and many dropped away and became distant. When Aiva was born I couldn't wait to take her out and show her off to the world. It made me realise that becoming a mother can be an alienating experience, and before you know it you don't want to leave the house unless it is to see the maternal and child health nurse or to get groceries. If you feel a bit like this, my advice is to take it slowly. Start with a walk around the block with baby in a pram (or in a sling) – the sunlight and fresh air will do wonders for your state of mind. As your confidence grows, you may decide to call your local council to find a playgroup, or some mother–baby activities, such as yoga, gym, dance or swimming.

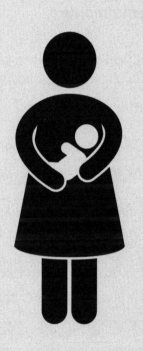

Most Aussies live within driving distance of some kind of waterway. If you are lucky enough to live not too far from a beach, it makes a wonderful day out, even with babies under 12 months.

- Grab an old fitted sheet to take with you and put a bag in each corner so you have yourself a nice little contained area.

- Make sure you take a beach tent, too (baby's skin burns easily).

- At lunch time, blow up a flotation ring and pop baby in it for an instant low-chair.

- Keep a paintbrush in the back of the car to quickly remove any pesky sand that might be stuck to the skin.

Explore your local parks. I know this sounds obvious, but have you checked out all the playgrounds and parks in your area? Make a list and try to go somewhere you haven't been before. Throw the scooters in the car and go exploring.

Check out discount websites, such as groupon.com.au or scoopon.com.au. You'll be surprised at what you can find at a fraction of the cost. For example, you might find a 50 per cent off deal for the entry fees to a play centre. The cinema is free for kids under 3 years, so find a kids' movie or head to a mums and bubs session. Water parks, theme parks, zoos, aquariums, animal sanctuaries and most other visitor attractions are free for kids under 3 years. Some private health insurance companies offer rewards for their customers that come in the form of discounted movie tickets and more. Make sure you do your research and find out what you are entitled to.

If you are out and about, it's a good idea to take your own lunches and snacks, as it can be very expensive to buy food. I will often pack a large lunch box for the quintuplets when I go out (most places don't mind). I usually make jam or peanut butter sandwiches for outings and I only do toppings such as cheese and ham when we are at home because I know it will be picked apart! I always try to be conscious of others who might have a nut allergy. I check with those around us if we are having a play date or I go for a safer substitute. Here are some great ideas for portable snacks and lunches:

Bananas
super easy to peel and
no packaging required!

Berries
when they're in season
and don't cost a
fortune!

Yoghurt
I fill reusable pouches from
a tub of good-quality
yoghurt (on special)

Cheese and crackers
(in separate containers)

Veggie sticks and hummus
(in separate containers)
cucumber, carrot, capsicum,
snow peas and steamed
broccoli all make great dippers

Hard-boiled eggs and
halved pitted olives

Savoury muffins
make a batch for the freezer
and take them out to thaw in
the morning

Homemade muesli bars
and bliss balls

Buy second hand and save your money for experiences! You can find so many treasures on eBay and buy and sell pages on Facebook. Some items are brand new and at incredibly low prices. The top five things I buy second hand are: sheets, cot blankets, clothing, shoes and toys. When buying household items, I always shop with a budget in mind, and I ALWAYS buy the generic brand if one is available. For example, home-brand cleaning products are so much cheaper and do the job just as well as more expensive branded products.

PLAN AHEAD. Most events set aside cheaper presale tickets that you can buy a couple of days before the official ticket sales. These are often available through your mobile phone carrier, car insurance company or simply check online. I recently took all eight of my children to a kids' carnival. The whole exhibition area was full of rides, and everything was covered under the $5 per child entry fee – a 50 per cent saving compared to door sale prices. Always plan ahead and do your research for upcoming events.

Start a festive fund. Beginning in January, with each grocery shop I buy a $15 voucher that can be used at multiple department stores. I know it doesn't seem like much, but over 52 weeks I accrue $780 to put towards gifts and/or food shopping for hosting a Christmas lunch. And unlike putting money in a shoebox on top of the wardrobe, I'm not tempted to spend it beforehand.

A Christmas tradition a few of my friends follow is to buy their children one thing in each of the following categories: something they want, something they need, something to wear and something to read.

Kids don't need a birthday party every year! I try to alternate the years with my eldest three, so they have to take turns as to who gets the party. For toddlers three and under, birthday parties don't need to be elaborate. If we're honest, they're really for the parents – an excuse to celebrate that they've managed to keep everyone in their household alive for another year!

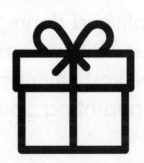

Keep parties simple. All you really need is a gift, a cake and a song. If you're not into baking, pressure to come up with a birthday cake can feel intense. If you want to give it a go, check out some of the cool cake hacks that bounce around social media. And when all else fails (and no one is dairy intolerant) grab an ice-cream cake. In my experience it will be demolished long before it melts. Try to relax and remember all you have accomplished during the year because, while you may not realise it now, you have smashed some major parenting goals!

AND DON'T FORGET TO TAKE PHOTOS.
In the newborn days, just the thought of photos can seem exhausting. But trust me, later down the track you will be so thankful you took the time to do it, especially when you look back at just how tiny and new they once were! When I had Aiva we didn't have enough money to have professional photos taken in a studio. I found a photographer in a Facebook group who was just learning the ropes of newborn photography and wanted to build her portfolio. I had some beautiful photos taken in the comfort of my own home, for free. Everyone has a camera on their phone now and it's easy to capture those memories. Be present with your little ones of course, but don't forget to take photos and videos, too.

Index

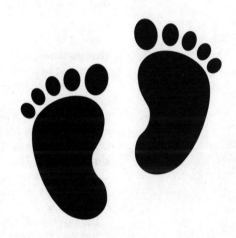

Acknowledgements

To my husband, Vaughn, thank you for always reminding me of my worth and supporting me through all of life's turmoil. I know you will always be in my corner if I need you.

Thank you to my family for all the support, love and encouragement this past year. It means more than I could ever say.

Thank you to Deborah Munson, who gave me a loving nudge and inspired me to write.

Most importantly, my children: I wouldn't be who I am today without all of you. Kurt, Aiva, Indiana, Tiffany, Keith, Beatrix, Penelope and Allison. I love you to the moon and back.

Last but not least, my two doggies, who have kept me sane and given me company throughout many hours of work on this book. I love you, Jem and Von!

To the talented team at Pan Macmillan, I can't thank you enough for all your support along this journey. I feel like I was given the dream team to help bring this book to life. My agent Pippa Masson, publisher Mary Small, editors Miriam Cannell and Ariane Durkin, and designer Alissa Dinallo: this book is just as much yours as it is mine.

First published 2020 in Macmillan
by Pan Macmillan Australia Pty Limited
1 Market Street, Sydney, New South Wales
Australia 2000

A CIP catalogue record for this book is available
from the National Library of Australia
http://catalogue.nla.gov.au

Text and cover design by Alissa Dinallo
Illustrations courtesy of Shutterstock
Author photographs by Erin Elizabeth Photography
Printed by McPherson's Printing Group

We advise that the information contained in this book does not negate
personal responsibility on the part of the reader for their own health
and safety and that of their family. It is recommended that individually
tailored advice is sought from your healthcare or medical professional.
The publishers and their respective employees, agents and authors are
not liable for injuries or damage occasioned to any person as a result
of reading or following the information contained in this book.

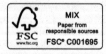